Amanda Medeiros Araujo de Oliveira
Tiago Silva Andrade
Belise M. O. Bezerra

Placental Efficiency and Calving Order in Pigs

Amanda Medeiros Araujo de Oliveira
Tiago Silva Andrade
Belise M. O. Bezerra

Placental Efficiency and Calving Order in Pigs

Correlating data to find better results

ScienciaScripts

Cover image: www.ingimage.com

This book is a translation from the original published under ISBN 978-3-330-99635-9.

Publisher:
Sciencia Scripts
is a trademark of
Dodo Books Indian Ocean Ltd. and OmniScriptum S.R.L publishing group

120 High Road, East Finchley, London, N2 9ED, United Kingdom
Str. Armeneasca 28/1, office 1, Chisinau MD-2012, Republic of Moldova, Europe
Managing Directors: Ieva Konstantinova, Victoria Ursu
info@omniscriptum.com

Printed at: see last page
ISBN: 978-620-8-59747-4

To myself, for my strength, courage and resilience.

ACKNOWLEDGEMENTS

To my parents: José Alves de Oliveira Sobrinho and Silvana Araújo Medeiros, for giving me the gift of life.

I would like to thank my boyfriend Danilo Batista Nogueira, a recent addition to my life, but one who has become very important.

My dog, Sofi, my great companion and confidante, especially during this last arduous year of university.

To my advisor Prof Dr José Nailton Bezerra Evangelista, who, as well as being a teacher, became a father.

To Prof Airton Alencar Araújo, for never refusing to help me.

To my friends Prof Marcio Araripe, Dr Camila Goersch and Dr Maurício Vieira for the knowledge they passed on to me with affection and all the patience in the world, and for having become a family within the university.

To my classmates, because we had unforgettable moments together.

To my supervisor Dr Tiago Silva Andrade, to whom I owe the credit for my passion for pig farming.

To the staff at the Xerez farm, especially Mr Givan, Carlão and Zim.

To the FAVET staff, Mr Marcos, Joélia, Dinho and Mr Alício, for all their help during the course and to all the people who contributed directly or indirectly to my graduation.

"It doesn't matter what you are, who you are or what you want. In life, daring to be different reflects on your personality, your character, what you are. And that's how **people will remember you one day."**

(Ayrton Senna)

SUMMARY

During pregnancy, various factors related to the uterine environment can influence foetal-placental development. Uterine vascular distribution, blood flow in the different regions of the uterus and even fetal location along the uterine horn are some examples of characteristics linked to conceptus survival and growth in hyperprolific species. Gestation in pigs lasts an average of 114 days, which can vary by up to four days depending on genetics, lineage, environment and management. This period is considered critical in pig farming due to its importance in developing individuals capable of achieving maximum productivity during their post-natal life. The aim of this study was to analyse the placental correlation with the birth order of the sows. 40 sows were used for the study and divided into four groups according to their birth order, so that there were 10 sows in birth order one, 10 sows in birth order two, 10 sows in birth order three and four sows in birth order four. Placental weights and litter weights were collected in order to calculate placental efficiency. According to the results obtained, birth order had no influence on placental efficiency, but other variables such as gestation length, litter weight and litter size had a direct influence. The weight of the piglet at birth is an extremely important factor, initially for its survival, and subsequently for good performance until the time of slaughter. Hyperprolific sows produce a greater number of piglets born per litter, which results in a lower average birth weight and, consequently, greater variability in the weight of these piglets. Therefore, traits such as placental efficiency and placental size should be included in genetic improvement programmes, as these aspects are seen as essential for producing more homogeneous piglets and, consequently, better viability.

Key words: Pig farming. Placental efficiency. Piglet weight.

SUMMARY

CHAPTER 1

DESCRIPTION OF INTERNSHIP CONDITIONS

The Compulsory Supervised Internship (ESO) was carried out in the areas of Production, Reproduction and Nutrition of Pigs and its objectives were to improve the knowledge previously acquired by the student during their degree and to monitor the practice of the Veterinary Doctor in their various areas of work, experiencing practices with ethics and professionalism.

This course conclusion paper refers to the compulsory supervised internship that took place at the company Xerez Avícola LTDA, based in the city of Maranguape - CE. It was carried out under the supervision of Ms Tiago Silva Andrade, the company's Veterinarian in charge of pig production, and under the guidance of Prof Dr José Nailton Bezerra Evangelista. The internship began on 01 August 2016 and ended on 31 October 2016, with a total workload of 526 hours.

CHAPTER 2

DESCRIPTION OF THE INTERNSHIP SITE

The Xerez Avícola LTDA company, located in the municipality of Maranguape - Ceará, has two Piglet Production Units (UPLs). The Tangueira unit (Figure 1) has 1419 sows and 14 boars. The Piroás unit has 600 matrices. This gives a total of 2019 breeding stock in operation, which characterises the company as a medium-sized farm when compared to farms in other Brazilian states. As for the Growing and Finishing units, the company has 10 properties located in the municipalities of Maranguape and Caridade, which together have a capacity for 20,000 animals for pork production. As the company is involved in intensive animal production, it operates 24 hours a day, with employees changing shifts.

Most of the internship took place at the Tangueira unit, where the company's Pig Reproductive Biotechnology Laboratory (LBRS) is located. The Tangueira unit, where most of the internship took place, has the company's pig semen laboratory. Semen doses are produced according to demand from the unit itself and also from the Piroás unit. There is also an accommodation shed for the males, together with the laboratory, a quarantine shed for receiving gilts, a collective gestation shed, four gestation sheds where the females are housed in cages, four maternity sheds with a capacity for an average of 70 sows with their respective litters housed per shed and three nursery sheds.

Xerez Avícola LTDA also produces poultry, with headquarters in the regions of Maranguape and Caridade, and a hatchery with a capacity of 95,000 eggs.

The pig and poultry production sectors are supplied by three feed factories, two in the municipality of Maranguape and one in the municipality of Maracanaú.

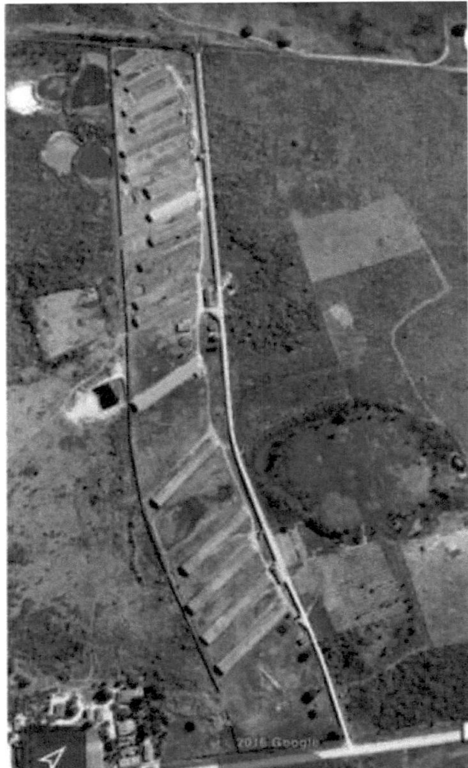

Figure 1 - UPL Tangueira facilities.
Source: Google Earth

CHAPTER 3

ACTIVITIES CARRIED OUT

The daily internship activities on the farm were carried out on working days, from 8am to 6pm, with a two-hour lunch break, totalling eight hours a day. As part of the internship routine, the professional's daily routine at the company was followed by visits to the UPL's and the Growing and Finishing Units (UCT), as well as visits to the farm's product suppliers.

The management applied in each production sector was observed in detail. As part of the learning process during the ESO, all the management observed will be described below. They were

observing the feeding of the animals; observing the cleaning and disinfection of the stalls and facilities (washing, fire broom and application of detergent/disinfectant); heat diagnosis accompanied by rutting; collecting, analysing and filling semen doses; artificial insemination; assisting with farrowing; castration of male piglets (normal and cryptorchid) and castration of old boars; necropsy to investigate cause of death in piglets and sows; weighing of animals; application of medication and dressings to animals; visits to feed factories; swine nutrition experiments (if interested); presentation and participation in talks for company employees.

The apprenticeship began in the LBRS. Afterwards, the Gestation, Maternity, Crèche, Growing and Finishing barns were observed and managed. Visits were made to the feed mills in order to observe the fundamental stages of the animal feed manufacturing process.

3.1PIG REPRODUCTIVE BIOTECHNOLOGY LABORATORY (LTRS)

The LBRS is extremely important and essential for the operation of the farm, as it needs a large number of piglets to establish itself. This large number is only possible if there is a satisfactory pregnancy rate. The method that makes this possible is artificial insemination. It was therefore decided that there was a need to follow the farm's laboratory routine in order to improve learning at this stage. On the farm, we found the basic equipment that allows the process of collecting, analysing, diluting and producing semen doses to function optimally. The room for receiving the collected semen was equipped with an oven, microscope, Neubauer chamber, semen filling equipment and a water bath. The storage room had a temperature-controlled fridge and the equipment to carry out reverse osmosis. In the collection room, there was a height-adjustable mannequin fixed to the floor, where the breeding animal was mounted, enabling seminal collection.

Collections were made twice a week to produce doses. If necessary, a new collection could be carried out with a minimum interval of two days. Daily checks were made to determine the quality of the semen doses prepared and stored.

Semen was routinely collected by a trained operator. A container was used, previously prepared by the laboratory manager, containing an isothermal cup and a beaker. A specific filter was placed over the opening to retain the gelatinous fraction. Collection was carried out using the gloved hand technique, in which the penis of the sire was gently pulled so that it was completely exposed. The animal's organ was placed next to the collection cup, which had been previously heated to 37°C, where the semen was deposited. At the start of collection, the first jets of ejaculate, which correspond to the pre-sperm fraction and are used to clean the urethra, were discarded. The objective at the end of collection was the rich fraction, containing 70% sperm cells, and the poor fraction, made up of seminal plasma and 30% sperm cells. All the procedures were carried out on the basis of the TOPIGS NORSVIN company manual®, which was also used to train the staff.

Immediately after collection, the ejaculate was taken to the laboratory, placed in a labelled beaker and placed in a water bath, so that the temperature was initially maintained and then gradually reduced to reduce the metabolism of the sperm cells.

Firstly, the volume of the ejaculate was determined. The presence of blood or urine was checked by staining. Then a microscopic evaluation was carried out, observing motility, vigour and agglutinations, using 100-200 times magnification and in three different fields. The sample was previously homogenised. A drop of the collected semen was then placed on a slide preheated to 35-37 °C. This was used to assess motility and quantify viability by observing the number of moving cells. This protocol is based on an evaluation of semen in natura, where samples with motility of less than 70% were discarded. The number of clumps of sperm cells, which are agglutinations, was observed. If there were more than 3 agglutinations per field, the ejaculate had to be discarded. At the Xerez farm, in order to determine the sperm concentration, which is a fundamental characteristic for calculating the number of inseminating doses, a direct cell counting method is adopted using a Neubauer chamber. After this count, the number of possible doses is calculated and the diluent is added, observing the cell concentration. The doses were filled in the laboratory itself and then stored under refrigeration at a temperature of between 15°C and 17°C, allowing them to be used for up to 3 days, which is when the loss of cell motility begins.

3.2PREGNANCY MANAGEMENT

3.2.1 Preparing gilts

The farm works with an annual replacement rate of 42 per cent, which means that the herd is constantly renewed throughout the year. That's why it was so important to take part in the observation of gilt management. It was noted that in order to achieve better reproductive planning on a commercial farm, it is ideal to have gilts of different ages. For example, if the farm received gilts that were 120 days old and 150 days old, the replacement management could be better programmed and the number and age of sows to be disposed of could be planned, introducing and disposing of sows on a regular basis.

With regard to vaccinations, the gilts received their first dose against Rhinitis seven days after arriving at the farm, and the second dose 15 days after the first dose. After 15 days on the farm, the gilts were also vaccinated against Circovirus and Mycoplasmosis. At 180-185 days of age, they were immunised with® Ery Parvo Leptoc as a preventative against Erysipelas, Parvovirosis and Swine Leptospirosis. The second dose was applied 15-20 days before the first immunisation. Pregnant gilts were given the vaccine against *Escherichia coli,* Rotavirus and Clostridiosis between the 70th and 76th day of gestation. The second dose was given on the 84th - 90th day of gestation.

The 120-day-old gilts received 2.5kg of feed a day. The 150-day-old gilts were given 2.0kg a day. When they reached 200-215 days of age, they were given 3.0 kg of Lactation type feed until the day of their first insemination, with the aim of maximising the ovulatory potential of these gilts. It was observed that the ambient temperature, health quality and weight of these females had an influence on feed consumption and, consequently, on the development of the gilts.

3.2.2 Multiparous

The multiparous and primiparous females were housed in gestation sheds, in individual cages with a trough-type drinker and semi-automatic feeder (Figure 2).

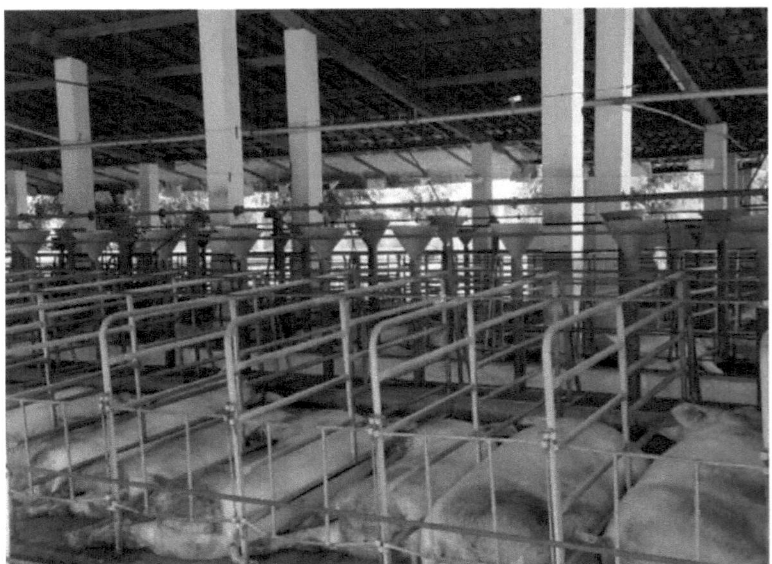

Figure 2-Gestation cages.
Source: Personal collection

On the farm, the sows were weaned after an average of 24 days of lactation. After weaning, the females went to the gestation sheds, where they were flushed and given 3.0 - 4.0 kg of feed until their first mating, facilitating the recovery of body reserves lost during lactation. This also facilitated the process of returning to heat, which took an average of five days.

Once inseminated, the sows were given gestation-type feed (2kg/day), fed once in the morning. Sows with a low body score received a total of 2.3kg/day, seeking better recovery and consequent success in the farrowing and lactation phase, with a high number of live births and a good piglet weight at weaning. During the final third of gestation, these sows were given pre-lactation type feed, with the aim of providing a better source of protein and vitamins, avoiding excess energy, as this is detrimental to the development of the mammary line due to the accumulation of fatty tissue in the mammary gland area. At this stage, there is a greater mobilisation of energy for the development of the piglets, as this is the period when the foetus doubles in weight.

The sows were vaccinated on the 84th - 90th day of gestation against Rhinitis, Escherichia coli, Rotavirus and Clostridiosis.

3.2.3 Oestrus diagnosis

The oestrus diagnoses were carried out in the presence of the ruffian male. The ruffian male was positioned in the corridors of the gestation shed between the cages where the sows were, subjecting them to the "Male Effect". This was done twice a day, in the early morning (6am) and late afternoon (5pm). While passing through the corridors, the ruffian had physical contact with the females, through snout-to-nose contact. When it was observed that the female showed signs of oestrus, such as immobility, an erect tail and ears, flushing and turgor of the vulva, a method was used to help with the diagnosis, which is the human tolerance reflex (HTR) (Figure 3). If the sow allowed this method, there was a further indication that she was in oestrus. Consequently, the sow that showed signs of oestrus was marked for later insemination.

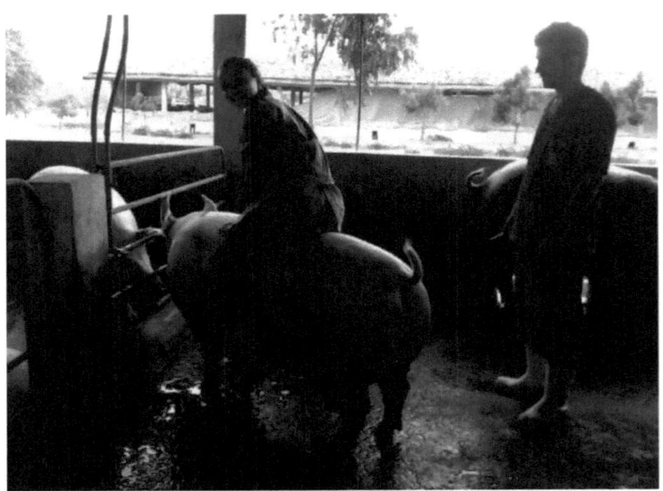

Figure 3- Tolerance reflex. Female showing signs of oestrus (motionless and with erect ears)
Source: Personal collection

3.2.4 Artificial Insemination

After adequate oestrus detection, the females were inseminated according to the insemination protocols adopted on the farm. Gilts were inseminated 00, 12 and 24 hours after oestrus detection. Sows were inseminated 12, 24 and 36 hours after oestrus detection. For example, when signs of oestrus were detected in a gilt, she was inseminated immediately afterwards. If the signs were observed in a multi-parent, insemination was carried out 12 hours after the first detection. When a female went into oestrus, a sequence of three inseminations was used at 12-hour intervals.

Another parameter to be followed was the difference between the type of pipette used. In gilts, the classic pipette pattern was used, which deposits sperm in the uterine cervical region, applying doses of 100 mL per insemination. In multiparous females, the intrauterine pipette was used, which deposits sperm directly in the uterus, with doses of 50 mL each.

3.3 MATERNITY MANAGEMENT

The sows were taken to the maternity sheds around five days before the day they were due to give birth. During the journey from one shed to the next, the sows were cleaned and disinfected. These movements took place during the most pleasant hours of the day, especially in the late afternoon.

In the maternity ward, the sows were fed four times a day, providing a quantity of 2 kg plus an additional 0.5 kg per suckling piglet (e.g. 12 suckling piglets = 8 kg (2 kg + 6 kg (12 piglets x 0.5 kg) of feed for the sow per day). Feeding was carried out during the cooler hours of the day, stimulating better consumption. If the sow had not yet given birth, only 2kg of feed was provided. And on the day the sow gave birth, there was no feed provided for this sow.

In order to facilitate and better control labour, a labour induction procedure was carried out with Veteglan® , which has a luteolytic effect. When administered, labour was expected to take place 24 hours after the administration of the hormone. This led to better planning on the part of the operators, providing adequate monitoring of the sow and the newborns. On the farm, this type of induction was only carried out on females that were beginning their 3rd gestational cycle, because when induction is carried out on 1st and 2nd calving females there is a greater risk of miscarriage. In this way, we avoided too many deliveries during the night and at weekends, when the number of operators was low.

After birth, each piglet was given its first care. Firstly, the neonate was dried with drying powder to prevent further heat loss or death by suffocation from the remains of foetal membranes and fluids. Next, the umbilical cord was tied off, cut and disinfected between 3 - 5 cm from its insertion with scissors and disinfected with 10% iodine tincture (Figure 4). Around 5mL of colostrum was provided through a syringe, guaranteeing a supply of antibodies during the first few minutes of life. Probiotic additives (Provitec® and Protexin(®)) were then given, providing immunity and energy for the newborn. After these procedures, the newborns were placed next to the teats and encouraged to suckle.

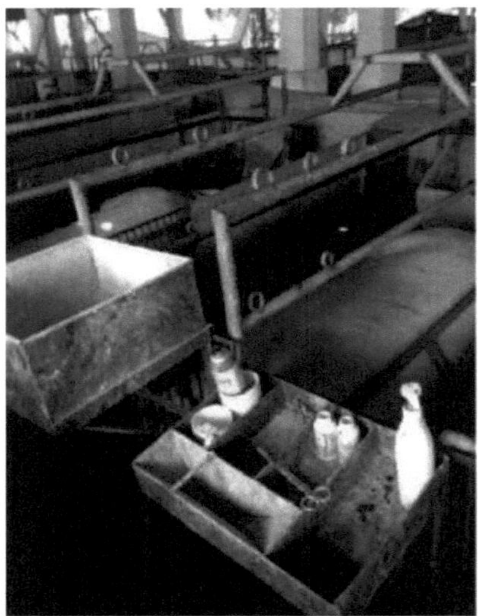

Figure 4- Material for first aid.
Source: Personal collection

In order to make labour easier, procedures such as administering iron, cutting teeth and trimming tails were carried out by the night shift operators. A few hours after farrowing, the litters were standardised to reduce competition for teats between piglets of different sizes.

The end of labour was characterised by the complete expulsion of the placenta. Normally, labour took place within a period of 2-4 hours. And the acceptable interval between one piglet being born and the next should be a maximum of 30 minutes. In dystocia, the time interval was

which required human intervention. Procedures were carried out to help the labour process, such as massaging the mammary glands and the abdomen in a craniocaudal direction with the hands, and massaging the mother's abdomen with the feet. This stimulated the mother's uterine contractions. The mother was also encouraged to stand up and lie down in the lateral decubitus position opposite the anterior side. Oxytocin was administered and, finally, the uterine touch was performed, with the piglets being manually removed from inside the vaginal canal. From then on, greater attention had to be paid to the sow's behaviour and general condition.

It was observed whether the sow resumed feeding normally, whether she was urinating and defecating properly, whether she was able to stand up and whether there was any vaginal discharge. With this, decisions could be taken to maintain or restore the sow's normal condition. In order to correct these problems, the administration of antibiotics (Norflomax®) for 3 to 5 days was recommended to eliminate the vaginal discharge. Glucose serum and/or the Herta Vita vitamin complex® were used to provide energy supplementation for the sow. In cases of anaemic sows, iron was administered.

Between the third and fourth day, more attention was paid to the newborn piglets. Farmacox® was given, which is a coccidiostatic antiparasitic that is essential for preventing coccidiosis diarrhoea in piglets. For the piglets that were not developing as expected, vitamin supplementation was administered, containing vitamins A, D, E and B12, so that they could regain muscle development.

At seven days old, the male piglets were castrated. The piglets were fed a type of feed that helps with the transition from breast milk to solid feed, so that they could get used to their future diet.

As part of the continuity of the sows' immunisation process, the vaccine® Ery Parvo Lepto was applied as a preventative against Erysipelas, Parvovirosis and Swine Leptospirosis when the sows were 12 days into their lactation.

During the week in which weaning took place, the piglets were given preventative medication (Zuprevo®) to prevent respiratory problems, which are common in the region due to the fact that the farm is located in an area with a hot and humid climate.

The piglets were weaned at 24 days of age. During this period, they received the first dose of the Circumvent vaccine® PCVM, as a form of prevention against Porcine Circovirus Type 2 and Mycoplasma hyopneumoniaye.

3.4 SCHOOL

The farm has 4 crèche sheds, which cover a total of 2900 piglets. It was observed that the animals entered the crèche at an average age of 24 days. The farm used a batch division system, where the piglets were distributed into three groups classified as batch heads (animals weighing more than 6kg), intermediate (animals weighing between 5 and 6kg) and batch ends (animals weighing less than 5kg). There was also a further batch where animals that fell ill or were not developing satisfactorily were grouped together for better monitoring and possible treatment. The aim of all this classification was to standardise the batch of animals so that there would be fewer disputes over feed, reducing stress and energy expenditure. It was found that this improved the piglets' weight gain, a factor that is characterised as the main objective of this phase.

During this period, the piglets had free access to the feed, which was provided in semi-automatic feeders, where the operators topped up the feed at least twice a day, so that there was always food available for the piglets (Figure 5).

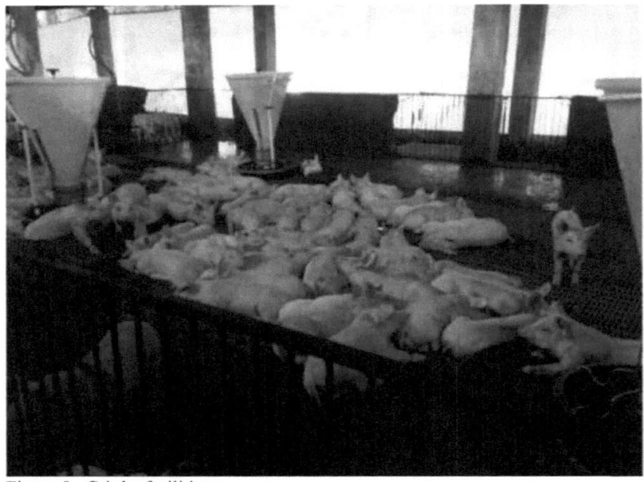

Figure 5 - Crèche facilities.
Source: Personal collection

The type of feed provided depended on the age of the animals. When they arrived at the crèche, the Pre-Start I type of feed was continued. For the head and tail animals, it was given for seven days, and for the intermediate animals, it was given for 10 days, in order to help them recover better. After the first seven days, the heads and ends were given the Pre-Start II ration, which was available for a further seven days. The intermediate animals, on the other hand, received this type of feed after the first ten days and would be available for a further four days. Thus, at the end of two full weeks, the three batches of animals were fed the Initial I ration. It was observed that from this stage onwards, consumption per animal increased considerably, as did the weight of the animals. This type of feed was given for a fortnight. After this period, consumption of starter II began, which was fed for a further two weeks.

At the beginning of the nursery phase, there was an incidence of diarrhoea, which can be explained by the stressful process of weaning. As a result, some measures were taken to combat and alleviate this problem. Injectable antibiotics and vitamin complexes were administered to the affected animals. We also used 350g of the antibiotic Neomycin in 1000 litres of water supplied to all the animals, which is a curative dose, but has a preventative effect on the other piglets that are not affected.

In these animals, a very common genetic problem of paternal origin can occur, which is cryptorchidism. Thus, during the normal castration process that was carried out in the maternity ward, it happened that one of the testicles could not be visualised because, due to the genetic defect, it was retained in the abdominal cavity. The procedure adopted to solve this problem was castration with a surgical incision made in the abdomen, close to the inguinal region. On the farm, this procedure was carried out on animals around 40 days old, because at this age it was easier and quicker to locate the testicles internally.

The piglets remained in this phase for an average of 42 days. They left the crèche when they were 63 days old on average and moved on to the growing and finishing phase.

3.5 GROWING AND FINISHING

During this phase, quick visits were made to check the zootechnical performance of the animals and to assess their management and environment. It was noted that this phase is characterised by intense preparation of the piglets, with the aim of weight gain, good feed conversion and good carcass quality. It was realised that the main factor determining success in these phases was nutritional management. The growth phase has the characteristic of requiring a denser feed formulation, with higher levels of energy and amino acids. Unlike the finishing phase, where these levels need to be reduced in order to reduce feed costs. Observing the zootechnical data, it was observed that there was a stabilisation in muscle development and a greater deposition of fat in the animal's carcass, showing that there was no need for a ration with an excessive number of additives and vitamins, which is what adds the most value to the ration.

As already mentioned, the company has 10 farms dedicated solely to growing and finishing animals. The piglets arrived at this stage at an average age of 63 days and stayed for a further 90 days on average. It was during this phase that the highest feed consumption was observed. The animals arrived weighing between 23-26kg and left weighing 90-105kg.

The feeders were filled twice a day, with the intention of feeding the animals ad libitum.

3.6 FEED MILL

The farm is supplied by three feed factories. Factory 1 is in the Amanari district and Factory 2 is in the Preá district, both located in the municipality of Maranguape. Factory 3 (Figure 6) is located in the municipality of Maracanaú. Due to the importance of the activity of a feed factory for a commercial farm, it was decided that visits and monitoring of the factory's routine would be essential. Visits were made to factories 1 and 3. Factory 1 produces the most feed, producing feed for all stages of the production system: Gestation, Pre-Lactation, Lactation, Pre-Initial I, Pre-Initial II, Initial I, Initial II, Growth, Termination and Male. The company also produced feed for the production phases of the poultry segment. During the visits, we monitored how raw materials such as corn and soya were received and how the material was stored, adopting measures to make the products viable for longer. For example, when receiving corn, a test was routinely carried out to check the maximum humidity limit allowed. When storing corn, the humidity in the room was controlled by painting the walls with copper sulphate. This reduced the presence of fungi and consequently the production of mycotoxins in the animal feed. An important stage in the feed manufacturing process was the weighing of the micronutrients needed to make up the feed, which was also carried out. The final mixing, manufacturing and pelleting process was also monitored. At factory 3, the visit was made to observe the soya extrusion process and to analyse the quality of the soya using the Urease test.

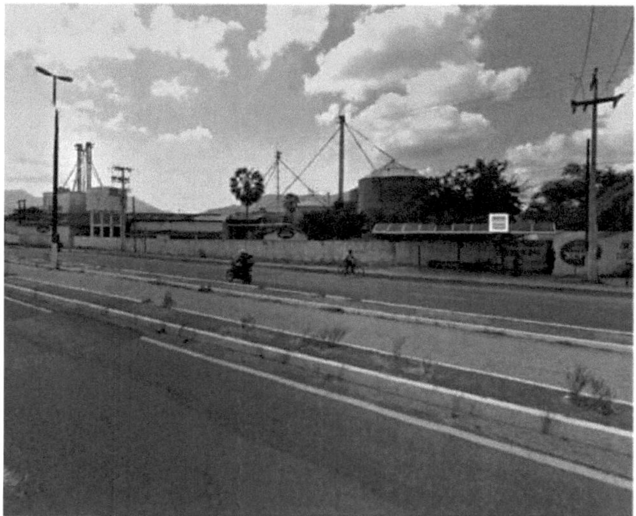

Figure 6-Facilities of Factory 1, located in the municipality of Maracanaú
Source: Personal collection

CHAPTER 4

CORRELATION BETWEEN PLACENTAL EFFICIENCY AND BIRTH ORDER IN PIGS

1 INTRODUCTION

Pig farming is an important segment of agriculture, responsible for generating millions of jobs worldwide and producing food. Pork is the most popular source of animal protein in the world, accounting for around 40% of all meat consumed, with a production of 104.363 million tonnes in 2012 (UNITED STATES DEPARTMENT OF AGRICULTURE - USDA, 2013).

In Brazil, pig production has undergone a great deal of development in recent years, thanks to the research carried out in the area and the high level of genetic gain in breeding stock. The increase in the technology used in pig farming has brought new challenges to the sector and, with them, the search to perfect the management practised, allowing for improved production efficiency.

The pig industry has focussed much of its attention in recent years on selecting highly productive sows, with the aim of increasing the number of piglets weaned per sow per year. Data from PIGCHAMP involving American herds has shown an increase of more than one piglet in the number of live births (10.2 vs 11.35) from 1998 to 2008 (FIX et al., 2010).In the Netherlands, the results indicated a steady growth of 0.35 piglets weaned/female/year, which leads to an estimate of 15 to 16 live births/sow or 33 weanlings/female/year by the year 2020 (SILVA, 2010).

In modern pig farming, success is largely related to the efficient reproductive performance of the sows. With the advance of genetic improvement, hyperprolific strains have emerged, resulting from the selection of highly prolific European strains or from crossing them with Chinese breeds, which are notoriously great piglet producers. However, with the increase in the size of the litter, many sows ended up producing piglets with low birth weights, a fact observed in the main pig producing centres. Piglets with low birth weights are more susceptible to disease, have higher mortality rates and compromised production performance, generating economic losses for the producer.

Sow productivity has increased over the years. In 1991, 1/3 of the best Canadian farms weaned 22.25 piglets/sow/year, a performance that, a decade earlier, was achieved by very few farms. With this productivity, it is possible to deduce that, a decade ago, the nutritional requirements of female pigs were different from those of today (PANZARDI, 2009). Considering that nutrient levels must be provided at each stage of gestation, failures in the production process can have variable consequences on the growth rate, the development of foetuses in the uterus, the weight of the piglet at birth, the body reserves themselves and subsequent performance. In the sow's productive cycle, reserves are only deposited during gestation and are highly dependent on the sow's metabolic status and intake of nutrients, especially amino acids, during this phase (CLOSE, COLE, 2001).

During pregnancy, various factors related to the uterine environment can influence foetal-placental development. Uterine vascular distribution, blood flow in the different regions of the uterus and even fetal location along the uterine horn are some examples of characteristics linked to the survival and growth of conceptuses in hyperprolific species. With the uterine overcrowding observed in pigs, these characteristics may be related to variation in conceptus development.

However, the intense selection pressure for ovulation rate has created an imbalance between ovulation rate, the number of conceptuses that survive the post-implantation period, placental efficiency and uterine capacity (FOXCROFT et al., 2009)

This leads to the birth of smaller, lighter and consequently weaker piglets, characteristic signs of what is known as intra- uterine growth retardation (IUGR) (FOXCROFT et al., 2006). These animals, affected by a nutritional deficiency while still in the womb, adapt to this deficiency through physiological and metabolic changes in order to increase their chances of survival after birth. However, these modifications, which occur at genome level, such as changes in DNA methylation, can remain throughout the animal's life, which is called prenatal programming (WU et al., 2004).

2 LITERATURE REVIEW

2.1 SWINE PREGNANCY PHYSIOLOGY

Gestation in pigs lasts an average of 114 days, which can vary by up to four days depending on genetics, lineage, environment and management (PANZARDI et al., 2007). This period is considered critical in pig farming due to its importance in developing individuals capable of achieving maximum productivity during post-natal life.

Normally, gestation in pigs is subdivided into thirds, the first of which is characterised by maternal recognition of the pregnancy and implantation of the embryos, while the second and third are characterised by foetal development (PANZARDI et al., 2007). Various genetic and environmental factors are responsible for the growth of maternal-fetal tissues during the gestational period, as well as for the variation in the number of piglets born.

During the first third of pregnancy, a series of events take place from the proliferation (cleavage) of the first cell originating from fertilisation (zygote) to the complete implantation of the conceptus and the formation of the placenta. The cleavage of zygotes follows almost immediately after the fertilisation process (HUNTER, 1977), occurring before the embryo reaches the uterine ostium of the fallopian tube, prior to entering the uterine horn. The cleavage process takes 2 to 3 days, when the organism has four cells. The morula stage (16-32 cells) is observed between the third and fourth days after ovulation, already in the uterus. This is followed by the formation of a fluid-filled cavity called the blastocele, which rapidly enlarges, giving rise to the blastocyst stage (HYTTEL et al., 2000).

The blastocyst is made up of a peripheral layer of large flattened cells called the trophoblast and an internal cavity, the blastocele, with a cluster of smaller cells next to the trophoblastic layer. The cluster of cells is called the inner cell mass (ICM), which gives rise to the embryo, while the trophoblast gives rise to the placenta and embryonic membranes (MILES et al., 2008). Between days 9 and 12, intrauterine embryo migration takes place to equalise the number of conceptuses per horn, making them fully occupied. Between days 12 and 16 of gestation, the porcine embryos begin to elongate, mainly due to the reorganisation of the cells, going from 4.0 mm to up to 1.0 metre in length. Elongation does not occur at the same time in all conceptuses due to an asynchrony in cell divisions and expansion between embryos (STROBAND; LENDE, 1990). This asynchrony, similar to what occurs during ovulation and fertilisation, results in embryos at different stages of development and can even lead to embryo death due to incompatibility with the uterine environment (GEISERT et al., 1990).

The establishment of pregnancy involves maternal recognition of pregnancy and implantation. Maternal recognition of pregnancy can be defined as the physiological process by which the conceptus signals its presence in the maternal system through the secretion of steroids, growth factors and cytokines, which act to prevent the secretion of Prostaglandin F2a (PGF2a), stimulate the secretion of proteins or act directly on the ovary to produce progesterone (GOFF, 2002), prolonging the lifespan of the corpora lutea (CLs). The progesterone produced by CLs acts on the uterus to stimulate and maintain uterine functions which are responsible for early embryonic development, implantation, placentation and successful foetus-placental development (SPENCER; BAZER, 2004).

According to Spencer and Bazer (2004), the endometrium secretes PGF2a regardless of whether the female is pregnant or not, but in pregnant animals, the conceptuses secrete estrogens, which in turn are anti-luteolytic. In non-pregnant animals, PGF2a is secreted into the uterine vasculature and transported to the CL to perform its luteolytic function and reduce progesterone production. In pregnant females, PGF2a secretion is exocrine and remains in the uterine lumen, preventing luteolysis. This hypothesis was supported by the high concentration of this hormone in the utero-ovarian vein between days 12 and 18 of the oestrus cycle in non-pregnant animals (GOFF, 2002; ZIECIK, 2002), which was not observed between days 12 and 25 in pregnant females (KILLIAN; DAVIS; DAY, 1976). PGF2a, when secreted into the venous system, is possibly transported by the countercurrent system from the uterine vein to the ovarian artery, binding to its luteal receptors (GOFF, 2002; ZIECIK,

2002).

In the process of maternal recognition of pregnancy, at least four embryos are needed to produce enough oestrogen to trigger the start of signalling (BAZER; THATCHER, 1977). Embryos initially synthesise oestrogen between days 3 and 6 of gestation (NIEMANN; FREITAG; ELSAESSER, 1989). However, it is between days 10 and 15 that the conceptuses produce enough oestrogen to trigger the initial signalling for maternal recognition of pregnancy (JAEGER et al., 2001). The second period of high oestrogen production occurs between days
These two phases of secretion are necessary to consolidate the prolonged exocrine redirection of PGF2a (SPENCER; BAZER, 2004). In addition, oestrogen also plays a role in the reduction of high-affinity PGF2a receptors in the luteal cells of pregnant animals between days 12 and 16 (GADSBY et al., 1993).

Prostaglandin E2 (PGE2) also plays an important role in maintaining pregnancy. According to Spencer and Bazer (2004), PGE2 competes for the same luteal receptors as PGF2a, protecting CLs from the luteolytic action caused by this hormone. In uninseminated sows, PGE2 is secreted around days 13 and 16 of the oestrus cycle, but three times less than PGF2a. In pregnant sows, PGE2 peaks earlier (days 11 to 12) so that it binds to luteal receptors before PGF2a is secreted. This author states that the PGE2:PGF2a ratio secreted by endometrial cells in pregnant sows is higher than in cyclic sows. The agent that most influences this ratio is oestradiol, which inhibits the PGE2-9-oxyreductase enzyme responsible for converting PGE2 into PGF2a, increasing the proportion of PGE2. Progesterone secretion is then stimulated by PGE2 and would be inhibited by PGF2a. Thus, the increase in the ratio of PGE2: PGF2a protects the luteal cells during the middle and end of the luteal phase against the inhibitory effects of PGF2a in terms of progesterone secretion (ZIECIK, 2002).

Implantation begins around days 13 and 14 of gestation through slight contact between the trophoblast and the uterine mucosa. Complete attachment occurs when there is an association between the uterine and trophoblastic microvilli, around day 18 (GEISERT; RENEGAR; TATCHER, 1982). From around gestational day 35, organogenesis is complete, with calcium deposition in the bones, thus beginning the foetal phase (PANZARDI et al., 2007).

During the foetal phase, already considered to be the middle third of pregnancy, the number of muscle fibres in foetuses is established, which is related to the efficiency of post-natal growth (DWYER; FLETCHER; STICKLAND, 1993). The development of these muscle fibres, as well as the fetal organs, takes place during this phase. In the final third of pregnancy, there is the greatest development of the mammary gland (76 to 90 days) and the most accentuated growth of the foetus (from 91 days) (FOXCROFT et al., 2006).

Throughout gestation in swine, up to 50% of embryonic and foetal loss can occur (WU et al., 2009). Although female pigs ovulate 12 to 30 oocytes, only 9 to 16 foetuses normally survive until delivery (TOWN et al., 2005). The first peak in embryonic death occurs between days 11 and 18 of gestation, i.e. in the peri-implantation period, with the majority of prenatal losses (> 75%) occurring during the first 25 or 30 days of gestation (FORD; VONNAHME; WILSON, 2002). Foetal losses that occur after the 30th day of pregnancy are the result of inadequate uterine capacity (WEBEL; DZIUK, 1974). Thus, successful establishment and maintenance of pregnancy requires hormonal communication between the mother and the foetus.

2.2 FOETAL DEVELOPMENT

As already described, the foetal phase begins when placentation is complete, organogenesis is complete and calcium deposition in the skeleton is observed at around 35 days of gestation (PANZARDI et al., 2007). Some studies have observed that the development of different foetal tissues occurs allometrically during gestation (SILVA et al., 2012).

As in other species, foetal growth in pigs is stimulated as gestation progresses, accelerating from the second half (KNIGHT et al., 1977). Mcpherson et al. (2004) observed that the weight of foetuses increases exponentially in relation to gestational age, being more pronounced during late gestation.

The nutritional supply provided by the placenta is closely related to cell proliferation and differentiation in foetal tissues. In pigs, the pre-natal development of some tissues, such as the intestinal epithelium and muscle fibres, can be considered a limiting factor in the animals' post-natal performance, with a future economic impact on production systems (FOXCROFT et al., 2009).

The process of intestinal development includes morphogenesis and the differentiation of the smooth intestinal mucosa into a tube lined with villi. According to Dekaney, Bazer and Jaeger (1997), the start of intestinal villus elongation is observed from 40 days of gestation in pigs. The prenatal phase is characterised by minimal stimulation of the gastrointestinal lumen (ZABIELSKI; GODLEWSKI; GUILLOTEAU, 2008). Before birth, the gastrointestinal tract is only exposed to small amounts of complex nutrients via the ingestion of amniotic fluid. It is also known that, at this stage, the rate of cell turnover and probably the rate of oxygen demanded by cell metabolism is much lower before than after birth (TRAHAIR; SANGILD, 2002).

The development of muscle tissue in pigs is essential for meat production. In mammals, the formation of muscle fibres (myogenesis) is restricted to prenatal development. Muscle fibres originate from myogenic precursor cells called myoblasts. These cells proliferate to form myotubes and eventually differentiate into muscle fibres (MCLENNAN, 1994).

Pigs are hyperprolific animals with a natural variation in birth weight, and this variation is strongly related to the number of muscle fibres present. Thus, piglets with a lower birth weight have a lower number of muscle fibres, which is due to a lower number of fibres that have differentiated during the period of prenatal myogenesis, due to various intrinsic and extrinsic factors (BERARD et al., 2010; DWYER; STICKLAND, 1991; TOWN et al., 2004; TSE et al., 2008). When this number of fibres is reduced, these piglets become less able to recover in terms of performance and weight gain in the post-natal period (GONDRET et al., 2005).

2.3 INTRAUTERINE GROWTH RETARDATION (CIUR)

Genetic advances in recent decades have increased the ovulation rate and, consequently, the prolificacy of pig sows, enabling some systems to produce more than

30 weaned piglets/sow/year. This change has created an imbalance between ovulation rate, the number of conceptuses that survive the post-implantation period and uterine capacity (FOXCROFT et al., 2009). In fact, an ovulation rate higher than the number of foetuses the sow is capable of carrying to term increases competition between foetuses for nutrients and oxygen. This leads to the birth of smaller, lighter and consequently weaker piglets, characteristic signs of so-called intrauterine growth retardation (IUGR) (FOXCROFT et al., 2006).

CIUR, which most commonly occurs in pigs, can be defined as a reduction in the growth and development of mammalian embryos and foetuses or their organs during gestation (WU et al., 2006). Before the 35th day of gestation, pig embryos are evenly distributed within each uterine horn and their weights do not differ considerably within each litter. However, after day 35, uterine capacity becomes a limiting factor for foetal growth even though the foetuses are relatively evenly distributed (BAZER et al., 2009). Blood flow rates and, consequently, the supply of nutrients to the conceptuses after the 30th day of gestation vary greatly along the length of the pregnant female's uterus (PÈRE; ETIENNE, 2000), due to differences in the structure and density of its vascularisation (FORD; VONNAHME; WILSON, 2002). The main consequences of CIUR for piglets are: lower birth weight and greater variability in piglet weight, which can result in lower neonatal survival, greater susceptibility to disease, reduced postnatal growth rate and poorer carcass quality at slaughter (WU et al., 2006).

Among the measures used to determine the occurrence of CIUR is foetal weight or birth weight of less than two standard deviations from the mean body weight for gestational age (WU et al., 2006). Prolonged foetal malnutrition causes a change in the metabolic rate of the foetus, with altered hormone production and tissue sensitivity to nutrients for energy supply. As a result, nutrients are stored in the form of fat and blood flow is redistributed to protect key organs such as the brain. Therefore, an animal affected by CIUR has smaller organs, with the exception of the brain, a phenomenon known as the "brain sparing effect". *Therefore, another* measure to determine the existence of CIUR is the ratio between the weight of the brain and the weight of the liver. In normal animals, this ratio is less than one. The occurrence of underdeveloped placentas may also be associated with CIUR, since placental weight and placental blood flow are correlated with foetal weight (TOWN et al., 2004).

In type II cases, asymmetric, inharmonious, expectant management will be restricted to maternal-fetal conditions and maturity. In adverse maternal situations (uncontrollable hypertension, severe haemorrhage) and fetal situations (anoxia), as well as when the fetus is mature, early delivery is essential.

With regard to aetiology, of the known causes, maternal arterial hypertension undoubtedly stands out as the main one, although there are still major difficulties in determining the different types of hypertension during the pregnancy-puerperal cycle. In this respect, Lin et al. emphasised that it is persistent hypertension, regardless of its etiology, which is responsible for impairing foetal growth. It should be added, however, that the etiology of hypertension is related to perinatal prognosis. Thus, it is the overlapping of pregnancy-specific hypertension with underlying hypertension that leads to the most serious disturbances in foetal growth.

2.4 UTERINE CAPACITY

A piglet's post-natal performance is directly related to its birth weight, which in turn is correlated to its ability to survive and develop in the uterine environment. Therefore, birth weight is an important economic characteristic for pig farming (QUINIOU; DAGORN; GAUDRÉ, 2002).

Embryonic and foetal development is a very complex and highly integrated process that depends on efficient communication between the uterus and the conceptus. Thus, the supply of nutrients to the conceptus and its ability to utilise the available substrates are essential factors for its development and depend on the available uterine space (REHFELDT; KUHN, 2006).

Uterine capacity is estimated by the number of conceptuses that the uterus can carry to birth, and its limitations are related to competition between conceptuses for uterine space and nutrient supply (FORD; VONNAHME; WILSON, 2002). It is characterised as a limiting factor for foetal survival between days 30 and 40 of gestation, when the placenta of each conceptus begins to expand rapidly, forcing it to compete for uterine space (FORD; VONNAHME; WILSON, 2002; VALLET, 2000). During this phase, the second highest foetal mortality rate is recorded (10 to 15%). The phase with the highest rate of conceptus loss (30 per cent) occurs in the peri-implantation period, between days 11 and 18 of gestation. Another critical phase occurs after 90 days, when mortality rates of 5 to 10 per cent are recorded, due to the peak in foetal growth which leads to increased competition for the limited uterine space (FORD; VONNAHME; WILSON, 2002).

Uterine capacity can also be defined in terms of the endometrial-placental bonding surface area needed to support the nutrient requirements of a foetus during gestation (FORD; VONNAHME; WILSON, 2002). Wu et al. (1989) determined the measurement of 36 cm of uterus per foetus as a requirement for implantation, survival and complete foetal development. Thus, uterus length becomes a limiting factor for litter size and piglet birth weight as the number of conceptuses increases.

In recent years, companies' breeding programmes have focused on productive and reproductive traits, such as feed conversion and daily weight gain of piglets, ovulation rate and litter size (LOVENDAHL et al., 2005), leaving traits such as uterine capacity, placental efficiency and maternal-fetal nutrition in the background. Johnson, Nielsen and Casey (1999), when reviewing the results of selection for litter size, concluded that genetic improvement programmes should better emphasise the variable "piglets born alive", since there are positive genetic relationships between ovulation rate and the number of stillborn and mummified piglets, and also because the relationship between birth weight and litter size is negative.

According to Ford, Vonnahme and Wilson (2002), in general, two factors seem to be involved in improving uterine capacity: the maternal effect and the individual effect of the conceptus. The maternal effect is related to the phenotypic characteristics of female pigs, which can provide greater space for the conceptus. The individual effect of the conceptus is related to the increase in placental efficiency due to the reduction in uterine space and, consequently, the size of the placenta. Within certain limits of uterine capacity, an increase in placental efficiency could initially protect the developing foetus from limitations in placental size (ALMEIDA, 2006).

Although there is information in the literature regarding fetal development, more studies are needed to understand this dynamic, contributing to future research into reproductive physiology and genetic improvement programmes.

2.5 . PLACENTAL DEVELOPMENT AND ITS RELATION TO FOETAL WEIGHT

The placenta is an organ formed by the juxtaposition of the embryonic trophoblast with maternal tissues inside the uterus. Placental tissue is highly vascularised by maternal and fetal vessels, and due to the proximity between them, allows for the diffusion of substances between maternal and fetal blood (DANTZER, 1985). The changes that occur in the developing placenta, altering vascularisation, are essential for cell growth and for the functioning of an effective gas and nutrient exchange pathway between mother and foetus (BERNARDI; WENTZ; BORTOLOZZO, 2006) and factors that stimulate angiogenesis are essential for maintaining good placental efficiency and thus ensuring good foetal development (ALMEIDA, 2009).

In pigs, the placenta is classified as epitheliochorial, diffuse and non-decidualised (BJORKMAN, 1973; DANTZER, 1985; RASHEV; GEORGIEVA; REES, 2005). The epitheliochorial placenta is made up of six layers of cells. These layers make up the foetal capillary endothelium, the foetal connective tissue, the foetal epithelium which is in apposition with the epithelium of the maternal endometrium, the maternal connective tissue and, finally, the maternal capillary endothelium (RENFREE, 1985).

In terms of the sites of attachment of the endometrium to the chorion, the porcine placenta is considered to be diffuse, since the microvilli of the chorion are evenly distributed over the entire surface of the chorionic sac. The placental microvilli attach to corresponding depressions in the uterine epithelium. Maternal-fetal exchange therefore takes place over almost the entire surface of the chorion (VALLET; MILES; FREKING, 2009).

The development of the placenta begins during the period of conceptus elongation, which is a key phase in controlling the size of the placenta. After elongation, the allantois develops externally to the embryo to form the chorioallantoic membrane, which defines the size of the functional placenta (VALLET; MILES; FREKING, 2009). During implantation, between days 14 and 16 of gestation, the cytoplasmic membranes of the trophoblastic and endometrial epithelia attach and adhere (MIGLINO et al., 2001). Implantation is the initial phase of placental membrane formation and placentation is complete around days 25 and 30 of gestation, with the development of interdigitations between the foetal and maternal microvilli. Between days 30 and 35 of gestation, the double layer made up of the trophoblastic and endometrial epithelia forms a set of microscopic folds (VALLET; MILES; FREKING, 2009). Fetal and maternal capillaries develop adjacent to this region and blood flows are organised in a counter-current transverse manner (LEISER; DANTZER, 1988; VALLET; MILES; FREKING, 2009). With the exception of nutrients secreted by glands, nutrient exchange takes place between these capillaries within the placental folds (VALLET; MILES; FREKING, 2009).

The uterine glands are numerous and have high secretory activity during pregnancy (BAZER; FIRST, 1983). Placental expansions develop over the opening of these glands to form the areola, an accessory structure made up of specialised cells with a high absorptive capacity that act in fetal histotrophic nutrition (WOODING; BURTON, 2008). The areolar lumen is rich in glycoproteins, one of which is involved in the transport of iron from mother to foetus, uteroferrin (MIGLINO et al., 2001), which is necessary for foetal haematopoiesis.

With these morphological characteristics described, it can be seen that the pig placenta is made up of interareolar subunits for blood exchange and areolar gland complexes used to transfer the large molecules that make up the histiotroph (BERNARDI; WENTZ; BORTOLOZZO, 2006). Neovascularisation of the developing placenta is essential for cell growth and to function as an effective route for gas and nutrient exchange between the mother and the conceptus. Various growth factors, such as IGF, TGF-p, PDGF, VEGF, are important for the growth and vascularisation of the placenta (DANTZER; WINTHER, 2001).

At 85 days of gestation, the placental folds deepen and become more complex, increasing the surface area. The double epithelial layer becomes less thick, increasing the proximity between the surface of each layer and the capillaries (VALLET; MILES; FREKING, 2009).

Knight et al. (1977) recorded an exponential increase in placental weight between days 20 and 70 of gestation, with little increase thereafter. However, a further increase in mass (approximately 25 per cent) has been observed between 90 and 100 days of gestation, with a significant increase in placental surface area between 100 and 110 days of gestation (BIENSEN; WILSON; FORD, 1998). An important component of placental function is the development of a sufficient absorption area, regardless of its physical size, but also the number and density of blood vessels for the exchange of nutrients (BERNARDI; WENTZ; BORTOLOZZO, 2006).

The uterine environment seems to determine placental size to a large extent up to 90 days of gestation (BIENSEN; WILSON; FORD, 1998; WILSON et al., 1998). After this period, the high demand for nutrients needed to support rapid foetal growth can occur through placental growth and the consequent increase in the surface area of maternal-foetal exchange, or by increasing vascular density and maintaining an almost constant placental surface. The results of studies carried out on the Meishan and Yorkshire breeds reinforce this idea. While the placentas of Yorkshire foetuses substantially increased in weight and length between days 70 and 110 of gestation, there was no increase in the weight or length of the placentas of Meishan foetuses in the last 40 days of gestation (BIENSEN; WILSON; FORD, 1998).

At the time of delivery, the placenta separates easily at the junction of the foetal and maternal microvilli and the incidence of retained placentas is insignificant in pigs. Hormonal changes, such as the release of relaxin from the corpus luteum from the increase in prostaglandins that trigger labour, are undoubtedly involved in the release of fetal and maternal tissues to allow easy placental separation (BAZER; FIRST, 1983).

2.6 PLACENTAL EFFICIENCY

In mammals, the main factor responsible for intrauterine growth is the supply of nutrients from the placenta to the foetus (FOWDEN et al., 2006). In fact, in many species, foetal weight close to birth is positively correlated with placental weight, as a proxy measure of maternal-foetal surface area for nutrient transport (BAUR, 1977; MELLOR, 1983). In turn, the placenta's ability to transfer nutrients depends on its size, morphology, blood flow and transport capacity (FOWDEN et al., 2006). In addition, placentation and the metabolism of essential nutrients and hormones influence the rate of foetal growth (FOWDEN; FORHEAD, 2004). Thus, alterations in any of these placental factors can affect intrauterine growth (FOWDEN et al., 2006; JONES; POWELL; JANSSON, 2007).

Placental function in nutrient supply is highly dependent on blood flow and maternal-fetal exchange area (SCHNEIDER, 1991), making the surface area available for endometrial placentation a critical factor in pre-natal survival (WRATHALL, 1971). The number, density and orientation of the capillaries present in this contact region determine the amount of nutrients that reach the foetus.

Placental efficiency is measured by the ratio between the piglet's birth weight and the weight of its placenta (WILSON; BIENSEN; FORD, 1999). A high placental efficiency would allow smaller placentas to maintain adequate foetal development without affecting viability (WILSON et al., 1998).

Meishan breed pigs have placentas that are more efficient at making nutrients available to the foetus due to greater blood flow, when compared to European and American breeds. Meishan placentas are smaller, but have an intense proliferation of blood vessels in the chorioallantoic membrane (BIENSEN; WILSON; FORD, 1998). As a result, this breed has higher embryonic survival, more numerous and homogeneous litters (WILSON et al., 1998), as well as a low percentage of stillbirths and a high survival rate from birth to weaning (HALEY; LEE; RITCHIE, 1995).

When analysing the placental weight of Meishan and Yorkshire piglets at 90 days of gestation and at farrowing, Wilson et al. (1998) found that placentas from Meishan foetuses showed similar weights both at 90 days and at farrowing. On the other hand, placentas from Yorkshire females showed an increase in weight of around 70 per cent from 90 days gestation to parturition. This shows that in Meishan females, placental blood flow is very important for the placenta to be more efficient in providing nutrients to the foetus. In this sense, adequate placental angiogenesis is critical for establishing placental circulation and maintaining adequate uterine and umbilical blood flow for normal foetal growth. Factors that influence aspects of the development and function of placental vascularisation can have a marked effect on fetal growth and therefore have consequences for neonatal survival and growth.

With regard to genetic selection, the heritability found for placental efficiency is higher than that observed for uterine capacity or the number of piglets born in total (VALLET et al., 2001). According to Wilson, Biensen and Ford (1999), sows selected for high placental efficiency had 3.3 more piglets/lactation than those selected for low placental efficiency (12.8 vs. 9.5 piglets). When evaluating placental efficiency in order to compare this trait in relation to birth weight and placental weight to predict the risk of pre-weaning mortality, Renset al. (2005) observed that placental efficiency is a complex trait to evaluate, since its effect on the risk of pre-weaning mortality is highly dependent on birth weight and placental weight, and of these two traits, birth weight is seen as the best predictor of the effect of placental efficiency on pre-weaning mortality (PANZARDI et al., 2007).

Genetic estimation of piglet survival values is positively related to placental efficiency (LEENHOUWERS et al., 2002). However, there is a limiting factor that is determined by uterine capacity, since birth weight increases in line with placental efficiency, but only until the conceptus reaches a maximum weight of around 1.6kg, declining thereafter (RENS et al., 2005).

3 MATERIAL AND METHODS

3.1 PROPERTY IDENTIFICATION

The experiment was carried out at the Tangueira Piglet Production Unit of the company Xerez Avícola LTDA, located in the city of Maranguape-CE. The UPL has a herd of 1,419 females and 14 cachaços for semen collection. Its facilities include an accommodation shed for the males along with a laboratory for making semen doses, a quarantine shed for receiving gilts, a collective gestation shed, four gestation sheds where the females are housed in cages, four maternity sheds with capacity for an average of 70 sows with their respective litters housed and four nursery sheds.

3.2 INSTALLATIONS AND EQUIPMENT

The maternity pens were arranged in an east/west direction and had Ductofan, an individual ventilation system for the lactating sows, where the air jet is directed towards the anterior region of the animal's back in order to provide better thermal comfort. They also used adjustable curtains on their sides to control the entry of draughts, especially at colder times of the day, as these draughts can be detrimental to the piglet's development. The maternity stalls are partially suspended, only part of the floor of the pen and the stall had a compact floor, the other areas had a hollow plastic floor, which favoured cleanliness, air circulation and the well-being of the sow and piglets. The stalls also had dummy-type drinkers at different heights and shell-type feeders for the sows and piglets.

3.3 ANIMALS USED

We used 40 females from the Topigs 20® commercial line from TOPIGS NORSVIN® , of different weights and ages. These females were allocated into four groups so that G1 (group 1) had ten primiparous females, G2 (group 2) had ten second calving females, G3 (group 3) had ten third calving females and G4 (group 4) had ten multiparous females with more than four births.

3.4 PERIOD OF EXECUTION

The study period was from 10 to 26 August 2016.

3.5 WEATHER CONDITIONS

The average values for the ambient temperature of the location where the experiment was carried out were observed, using data from the meteorological website Climate-data.org (2016), in order to know the temperature variation of the location (Maranguape-CE).

3.6 MANAGEMENT

The females in groups 1, 2, 3 and 4 were monitored throughout labour to obtain placental and litter weights, which made it possible to calculate the placental efficiency of each animal. As all the females were identified, this made it possible to correlate the placental efficiency of each female with her calving order.

3.6.1 Monitoring childbirth

All the sows were monitored during the farrowing process and the newborn piglets were cared for according to the farm's protocol. Sows that required any kind of assistance, such as touch or medication, were duly identified.

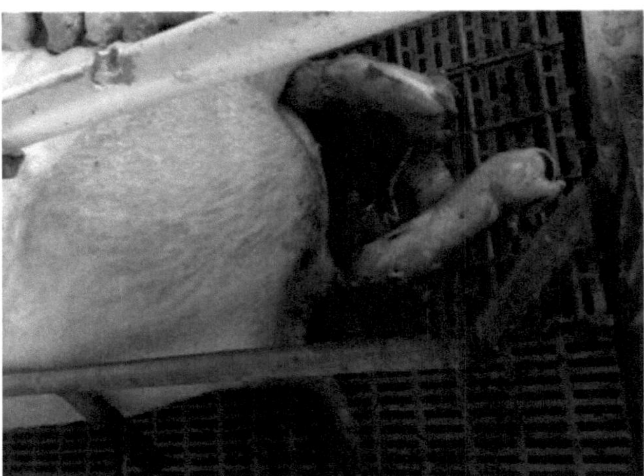

Figure 7-Moment of farrowing (piglets and placenta in the maternity pen)

Source: Personal collection

3.6.2 Weighing the placentas

The placentas were collected immediately after their expulsion along with the umbilical cord and weighed on a precision scale. These weighings took place throughout the labour process to avoid bias due to the evaporation of liquids if the material was kept for later weighing.

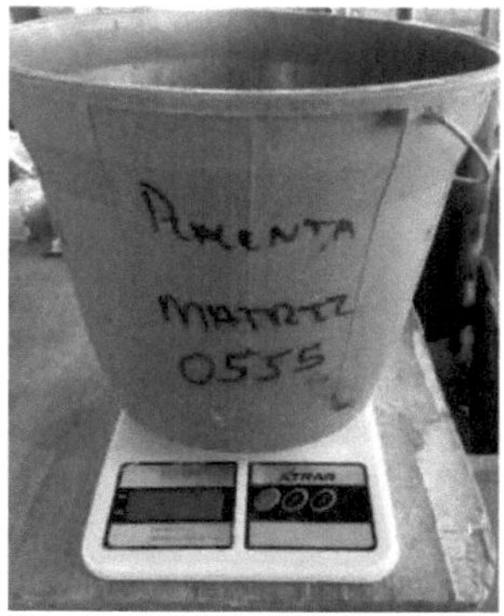

Figure 8 - Buckets containing placenta at the time of weighing.
Source: Personal collection

3.6.3 Weighing the piglets

All the piglets were weighed individually immediately after giving birth.

3.7 CALCULATING PLACENTAL EFFICIENCY

Two variables were used to calculate placental efficiency (CEP): one was total litter weight (PTL), calculated by adding up the weights of piglets born alive, stillborn, mummified and macerated, and the other was placental weight (PP). The ratio between PTL and PP results in a number that indicates the placental efficiency of the sow analysed.

3.8 STATISTICS

Analyses of variance were carried out using the GLM procedure and Pearson's correlations using the CORR procedure, both in the SAS statistical programme (SAS, Inst., Inc., Cary, NC).

4 RESULTS AND DISCUSSION

According to the results found in this study, with a sample of 40 females, there was no significant influence of calving order on placental efficiency. However, it was possible to identify a high relationship between gestation length and calving order, as can be seen in Graph 1.

Duração da gestação

■ M.A. ■ DM

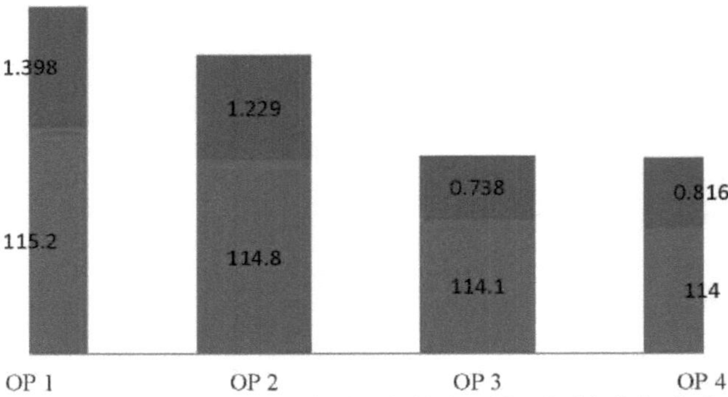

Graph 1-Arithmetic mean of gestation length (blue) and Standard deviation (red)
Source: Prepared by the author

At the end of gestation, foetal weights were higher than those reported more than a decade ago by Leenhouwers et al. (2002). This is an indication that there has been an improvement in foetal growth in recent years, mainly due to the selection of female pig lines aimed at high reproductive performance and with high prolificacy (BURRIN, 2001; POND;MERSMANN, 2001), capable of producing animals with higher birth weights, as well as maintaining colostrum and milk production during the lactation period.

There was a positive correlation between Placental Efficiency and Lactation Weight, showing that the healthy development of the placenta during the gestation period guarantees the development of a sufficient absorption area for the foetuses inside the uterus, which makes their development possible. According to graph 2, only females from Calving Order 1 did not achieve the expected result when comparing placental efficiency and litter weight, which is mainly due to the fact that the animal is still in the growth phase, which limits its uterine capacity.

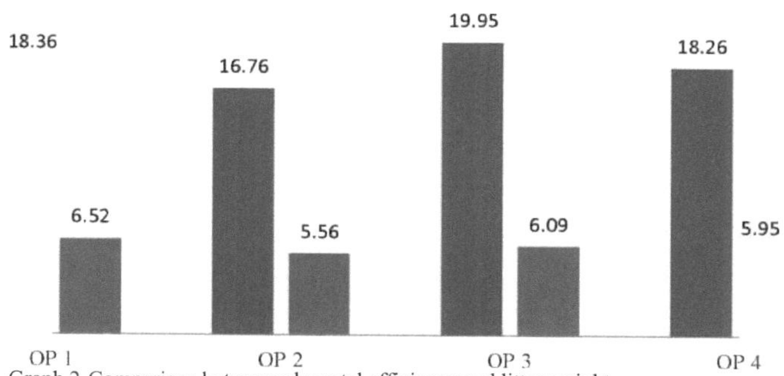

Graph 2-Comparison between placental efficiency and litter weight
Source: Prepared by the author

Contrary to what is usually reported in the literature regarding the effect of litter size on birth weight (Graph 3) (BEAULIEU et al., 2010; BERARD; KREUZER; BEE, 2008), a positive correlation was observed between the number of foetuses and the growth and average weight of the piglet, although the uterine capacity acts as a limiting factor for embryonic growth (FORD; VONNAHME; WILSON, 2002). Some tissue growth factor produced by the conceptuses themselves may be acting significantly on these genetics, but this could not be proven with the data from the present study.

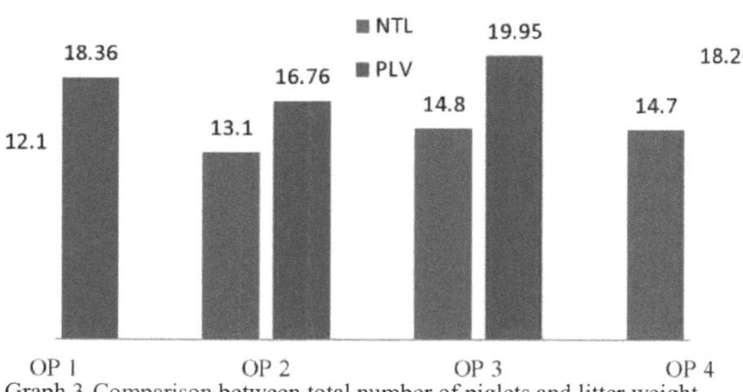

Graph 3-Comparison between total number of piglets and litter weight
Source: Prepared by the author

As reported in other studies (VALLET; FREKING, 2007; WISE; ROBERTS; CHRISTENSON, 1997), placental weights were lower in lighter litters and higher in heavier litters in all the calving orders studied.

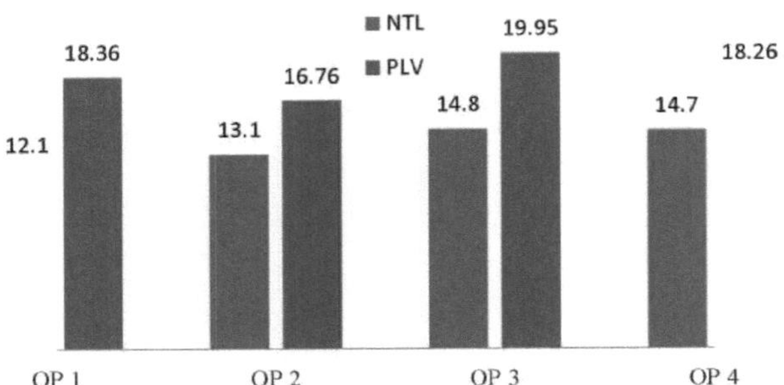

Graph 4-Demonstration of average litter size for each calving order and their respective total piglet weight

Source: Prepared by the author

The results of this study open the way for further research into the mechanisms and factors involved in foetal development in pigs, especially with regard to uterine capacity and placental efficiency. The discovery

of the main growth factors involved and their mechanisms of action in both the placenta and foetuses could help in nutrition and genetic improvement research aimed at producing even more prolific pig sows.

CHAPTER 5

CONCLUSION

In view of the above, it has been measurably observed that the farrowing order of the sow does not influence placental efficiency, but it can have an effect on other variables such as gestation length and litter weight. The weight of the piglet at birth is an extremely important factor, initially for its survival, and subsequently for good performance up to the time of slaughter. Hyperprolific sows produce a greater number of piglets born per litter, which results in a lower average birth weight and, consequently, greater variability in the weight of these piglets. Uterine capacity is a limiting factor in this respect, as it is a trait that has previously been exploited in breeding processes in an attempt to increase litter size. Therefore, traits such as placental efficiency and placenta size should be included in breeding programmes, as they are seen as essential aspects for producing more homogeneous piglets and, consequently, better viability. Nutrition and feed management, meanwhile, must be carried out thoroughly, always respecting the different reproductive phases that the sows are in, in order to provide high nutritional quality and thus a good piglet weight at birth. These two associated factors, genetics and nutrition, will certainly help to increase piglet survival during the lactation phase, thereby making a positive contribution to reducing the mortality rate in the maternity ward and increasing the economic gain from production.

REFERENCES

ALMEIDA, F. R. C. L. Influence of sow nutrition on piglet quality at birth. Acta Scientiae Veterinariae, Porto Alegre, v. 37, n. 1, p. 31-33, May 2009. Supplement.

ALMEIDA, F. R. C. L. Embryonic mortality and uterine capacity: factors determining litter size. In: SIMPÓSIO INTERNACIONAL DE PRODUÇÃO SUÍNA, 2., 2006, Campinas. Proceedings... Campinas: Consuitec, 2006. p. 109-115.

BAZER, F. W. et al. Comparative aspects of implantation. Reproduction, Cambridge, v. 138, n. 3, p. 195-209, Sept. 2009.

BAZER, F. W.; FIRST, N. L. Pregnancy and parturition.Journal of Animal Science, Champaign, v. 57, p. 425-460, 1983.

BAZER, F. W.; THATCHER, W. W. Theory of maternal recognition of pregnancy in swine based on estrogen controlled endocrine versus exocrine secretion of prostaglandin F2alpha by the uterine endometrium. Prostaglandins, Sheffield, v. 14, p. 397-400, 1977.

BERARD, J. et al. Intrauterine crowding decreases average birth weight and affects muscle fibre hyperplasia in piglets. Journal of Animal Science, Champaign, v. 88, n. 10, p. 3242-3250, Oct. 2010.

BERNARDI, M. L.; WENTZ, I.; BORTOLOZZO, F. P. Development of the porcine conceptus and factors predisposing to mummification. In: UFRGS SYMPOSIUM ON SWINE PRODUCTION, REPRODUCTION AND HEALTH, 1., 2006, Porto Alegre. Proceedings...Porto Alegre: UFRGS, 2006. p. 236-250.

BIENSEN, N. J.; WILSON, M. E.; FORD, S. P.The impact of either a Meishan or Yorkshire uterus on Meishan or Yorkshire foetal and placental development to days 70, 90 and 110 of gestation. Journal of Animal Science, Champaign, v. 76, n. 8, p. 2169-2176, Aug. 1998.

BJORKMAN, N. Fine structure of the fetalmaternal area of exchange in the epitheliochorial and endotheliochorial types of placentation. Acta Anatomy, Basel, v. 61, p. 1-22, 1973.

CLOSE, W.H. & COLE, D.J.A. 2001.Nutrition of sows and boars.1.ed.Nottinghan: Nottinghan University Press, 377p.

DEKANEY, C. M.; BAZER, F. W.; JAEGER, L. A. Mucosal morphogenesis and city of differentiation in foetal porcine small intestine. The Anatomical Record, New York, v. 249, n. 4, p. 517-523, Dec. 1997.

DWYER, C. M.; FLETCHER, J. M.; STICKLAND, N. C. Muscle cellularity and postnatal growth in the pig. Journal of Animal Science, Champaign, v. 71, n. 12, p. 3339-3343, Dec. 1993.

FIX, J.S.; CASSADY, J.P.; HERRING, W.O.; HOLL, J.W.; CULLBERTSON, M.S.; SEE, M.T. Effect of piglet birth weight on body weight, growth, backfat, and longissimus muscle area of commercial market swine. Livestock Science, v.127, p.51-59, 2010.

FOWDEN, A. L. et al. Programming placental nutrient transfer capacity. Journal of Physiology, Cambridge, n. 572, p. 5-15, 2006.

FOWDEN, A. L.; FORHEAD, A. J. Endocrine mechanisms of intrauterine programming. Reproduction, Cambridge, v. 127, n. 5, p. 515-526, May 2004.

FORD, S. P.; VONNAHME, K. A.; WILSON, M. E. Uterine capacity in the pig reflects a combination of uterine environment and conceptus genotype effects. Journal of Animal Science, Champaign, v. 80, n. 1, p. 66-73, Jan. 2002.

FOXCROFT, G. R. et al. The biological basis for prenatal programming of postnatal performance in pigs. Journal of Animal Science, Champaign, v. 84, n. 13, p. 105-112, Apr. 2006.

FOXCROFT, G. R. & TOWN, S. 2009. Prenatal programming of postnatal performance - The unseen cause of variance.Advanced Pork Production. v. 15, p. 269-279.

GADSBY, J. E. et al. Prostagladin F2 receptor concentrations in corpora lutea of cycling, pregnant, and pseudopregnant pigs. Biology of Reproduction, Champaign, v. 49, n. 3, p. 604-608, Sept. 1993.

GEISERT, R. D. et al. Embryonic steroids and the establishment of pregnancy in pigs. Journal of Reproduction and Fertility, Cambridge, n. 40, p. 293-305, Apr. 1990. Supplement.

GOFF, A. K. Embryonic signals and survival. Reproduction in Domestic Animals, Belfast, v. 37, n. 3, p. 133-139, June 2002.

GONDRET, F. et al. Influence of piglet birth weight on postnatal growth performance, tissue lipogenic capacity and muscle histological traits at market weight. Livestock Production Science, Amsterdam, v. 93, n. 2, p. 137-146, Nov. 2005.

HALEY, C. S.; LEE, G. L.; RITCHIE, M. Comparative farrowing to weaning performance in Meishan and Large White pigs and crosses. Animal Science, Edinburgh, v. 60, n. 2, p. 259-267, Oct. 1995.

HUNTER, R. H. F. Physiological factors influencing ovulation, fertilisation, early embryonic development and establishment of pregnancy in pigs. British Veterinary Journal, London, v. 133, p. 461-470, 1977.

HYTTEL, P. et al. Nucleolar proteins and ultrastructure in preimplantation porcine embryos developed in vivo. Biology of Reproduction, Champaign, v. 63, n. 6, p. 1848-1856, Dec. 2000.

JAEGER, L. A. et al. Functional analysis of autocrine and paracrine signalling at the uterine-conceptus interface in pigs.Reproduction, Cambridge, n. 58, p. 191-207, 2001. Supplement.

JOHNSON, R. K.; NIELSEN, M. K.; CASEY, D. S. Responses in ovulation rate, embryonic survival, and litter traits in swine to 14 generations of selection to increase litter size. Journal of Animal Science, Champaign, v. 77, n. 3, p. 541-557, Mar. 1999.

JONES, H. N.; POWELL, T. L.; JANSSON, T. Regulation of placental nutrient transport: a review. Placenta, London, v. 28, n. 8/9, p. 763-774, Aug./Sept. 2007.

KILLIAN, D. B.; DAVIS, D. L.; DAY, B. N. Plasma PGF and hormonal changes during the estrous cycle and early pregnancy in the gilt. In: INTERNATIONAL PIG VETERINARY SOCIETY, 1., 1976, Ames. Proceedings. Ames: IPVS, 1976. 1 CD-ROM.

KNIGHT, J. W. et al. Conceptus development in intact and unilaterally hysterectomised- ovariectomized gilts: Interrelations among hormonal status, placental development, fetal fluids and fetal growth. Journal of Animal Science, Champaign, v. 44, p. 620-637, 1977.

LEENHOUWERS, J. I. et al. Fetal development in the pig in relation to genetic meri for piglet survival.Journal of Animal Science, Champaign, v. 80, n. 7, p. 1759-1770, July 2002.

LEISER, R.; DANTZER, V. Structural and functional aspects of porcine placental microvasculature.Anatomy and Embryology, Berlin, v. 177, p. 409-419, 1988.

LOVENDAHL, P. et al. Aggressive behaviours of sows at mixing and maternal behaviour are heritable and genetically correlated traits. Livestock Production Science, Amsterdam, v. 93, n. 1, p. 73-85, Apr. 2005.

MCLENNAN, I. S. Neurogenic and myogenic regulation of skeletal muscle formation: a critical re-evaluation. Progress in Neurobiology, Oxford, v. 44, n. 2, p. 119-140, Oct. 1994.

MIGLINO, M. A. et al. Placental amorphology in domestic pigs. Arquivos de Ciências Veterinárias e Zoologia, Umuarama, v. 4, n. 1, p. 71-76, 2001.

MILES, J. R. et al. Conceptus development during blastocyst elongation in lines of pigs selected for increased uterine capacity or ovulation rate. Journal of Animal Science, Champaign, v. 86, n. 9, p. 2126-2134, Sep. 2008.

NIEMANN, H.; FREITAG, M.; ELSAESSER, F.The role of estrogens in early embryonic development.Journal of Reproduction and Fertility, Cambridge, v. 38, p. 73-83, 1989.

PANZARDI, A. et al. Chronological events of pregnancy: from the deposition of spermatozoa in the female reproductive tract to the development of foetuses. In: Pig farming in action: the pregnant pig. 4. ed. Porto Alegre: UFRS, 2007. p. 43-71.

PANZARDI, A.; BIERHALS, T.; MELLAGI, A.P.G.; BERNARDI, M.L.; BORTOLOZZO, F.P. & WENTZ, I. 2009. Survival of piglets according to physiological parameters at birth. In: Proceedings of the 8th International Conference on Pig Reproduction(Banff, Canada).

PÈRE, M. C.; ETIENNE, M. Uterine blood flow in sows: effects of pregnancy stage and litter size. Reproduction Nutrition Development, Paris, v. 40, n. 4, p. 369-382, July/Aug. 2000.

QUINIOU, N.; DAGORN, J.; GAUDRÉ, D. **Variation of piglets' birth weight and** consequences on subsequent performance. Livestock Production Science, Amsterdam,v. 78, n. 1, p. 63-70, Nov. 2002.

REHFELDT, C.; KUHN, G. Consequences of birth weight for postnatal growth performance and carcass quality in pigs as related to myogenesis. Journal of Animal Science, Champaign, v. 84, n. 13, p. 113-123, Apr. 2006. Supplement.

RENFREE, M. B. Implantation and placentation. In: AUSTIN, C. R.; SHORT, R. V. (Ed.). Reproduction in mammals: embryonic and foetal development. Cambridge:

Cambridge University, 1985, p. 26-69.

RENS, B. T. T. M. van et al. Preweaning piglet mortality in relation to placental efficiency. Journal of Animal Science, Champaign, v. 83, n. 1, p. 144-151, Jan. 2005.

SCHNEIDER, H. The role of the placenta in nutritionof the human foetus. American Journal of Obstetrics and Gynecology, Saint Louis, v. 164, n. 4, p. 967-973, Apr. 1991.

SILVA, B. Nutrition of swine sows with high reproductive performance in the tropics. In: SIMPÓSIO INTERNACIONAL DE PRODUÇÃO SUÍNA, 2010, Campinas/SP. Proceedings...Campinas, 2010.

SILVA, P. F. N. et al. Changes in the relationship between porcine foetal size and organ development during pregnancy. Available at:<http://lib.znate.ru/docs/index- 34319.html?page=18>. Accessed on: 10 August 2016.

SPENCER, T. E.; BAZER, F. W. Conceptus signals for establishment and maintenance of pregnancy. Reproductive Biology and Endocrinology, London, v. 49, n. 2, p. 1-15, July 2004.

STROBAND, H. W. J.; LENDE, T. Embryonic and uterine development during early pregnancy in pigs. Journal of Reproduction and Fertility, Cambridge, n. 40, p. 261-277, Apr. 1990. Supplement.

TOWN, S. C. et al. Embryonic and foetal development in a commercial dam-line genotype. Animal Reproduction Science, Amsterdam, v. 85, n. 3/4, p. 301-316, Feb. 2005

TOWN, S. C. Number of conceptuses in utero affects porcine foetal muscle development.
Reproduction, Cambridge, v. 128, n. 1, p. 443-454, Oct. 2004.

TRAHAIR, J. F.; SANGILD, P. T. Structural development of the foetalgastrointestinal tract. In: ZABIELSKI, R. et al. (Ed.). Biology of the small intestine in growing animals. Amsterdam: Elsevier, 2002. p. 1-54.

UNITED STATES DEPARTMENT OF AGRICULTURE. Data and statistics. Washington, 2013.

Available at: <http://www.usda.gov/wps/portal/usda/usdahome>. Accessed on: 3 April 2016.

VALLET, J. L. Fetal erythropoiesis and other factors which influence uterine capacity in swine. Journal of Applied Animal Research, Izatnagar, v. 17, n. 1, p. 126, Feb. 2000.

VALLET, J. L. et al. Are haematocrit and placental selection tools for uterinecapacity in swine?Journal of Animal Science, Champaign, v. 79, p. 64-73, Dec. 2001. Supplement 2.

VALLET, J. L.; MILES, J. R.; FREKING, B. A. Development of the pig placent.Society for Reproduction and Fertility, Colchester, n. 66, p. 265-279, Dec. 2009. Supplement.

WEBEL, S. K.; DZIUK, P. J. Effect of stage of gestation and uterine space on prenatal survival in the pig.Journal of Animal Science, Champaign, v. 38, p. 960-963, 1974.

WILSON, M. E.; BIENSEN, N. J.; FORD, S. P. Novel insight into the control of litter size in pigs, using placental efficiency as a selection tool. Journal of Animal Science, Champaign, v. 77, n. 7, p. 1654-1658, July 1999.

WILSON, M. E. et al. Development of Meishan and Yorkshire littermateconceptuses in either a Meishan or Yorkshire uterine environment to day 90 ofgestation and to term. Biology of Reproduction, Champaign, v. 58, n. 4, p. 905-910, Apr. 1998.

WOODING, P.; BURTON, G. Comparative placentation: structures, functions and evolution. Heidelberg: Springer Verlag, p. 314, 2008.

WRATHALL, A. E. Prenatal survival in pigs: part 1, ovulation rate and itsinfluence on prenatal survival and litter size in pigs. Farnham Royal: Commonwealth Agricultural Bureaux, p. 108, 1971 (Review Series, 9).

WU, G. et al. Amino acid composition of the foetal pig. Journal of Nutrition, Philadelphia, v. 129, n. 5, p. 1031-1038, May 1999.

WU, G. et al. Impacts of amino acid nutrition on pregnancy outcome in pigs: mechanisms and implications for swine production. Journal of Animal Science, Champaign, v. 88, n. 13, p. 195-204, Apr. 2009.Supplement.

WU, G. et al. Intra-uterine growth retardation: implications for the animal sciences. Journal of Animal Science, Champaign, v. 84, n. 9, p. 2316-2337, Sept. 2006.

WU, M. C. et al. Effect of initial length of uterusper embryo on foetal survival and development in the pig. Journal of Animal Science, Champaign, v. 67, p. 1767-1772, 1989.

ZABIELSKI, R.; GODLEWSKI, M. M.; GUILLOTEAU, P. Control of development of gastrointestinal system in neonates. Journal of Physiology and Pharmacology, Birmingham, v. 59, n. 1, p. 35-54, 2008.

ZIECIK, A. J. Old, new and newest concepts of inhibition of lutolysis during early pregnancy in pig. Domestic Animal Endocrinology, Auburn, v. 23, p. 265-275, 2002.

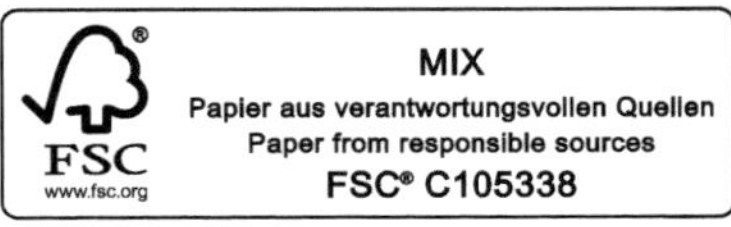

Printed by Books on Demand GmbH, Norderstedt / Germany